D1050536

Disclaimer

Medicine and nursing are continuously changing practices. The author and publisher have reviewed all information in this book with resources believed to be reliable and accurate and have made every effort to provide information that is up to date with best practices at the time of publication. Despite our best efforts we cannot disregard the possibility of human error and continual changes in best practices the author, publisher, and any other party involved in the production of this work can warrant that the information contained herein is complete or fully accurate. The author, publisher, and all other parties involved in this work disclaim all responsibility from any errors contained within this work and from the results from the use of this information. Readers are encouraged to check all information in this book with institutional guidelines, other sources, and up to date information. For up to date disclaimer information please visit: http://www.nrsng.com/about.

NCLEX®, NCLEX®-RN ®are registered trademarks of the National Council of State Boards of Nursing, INC. and hold no affiliation or support of this product.

All Rights Reserved. No part of this publication may be reproduced in any form or by any means, including scanning, photocopying, or otherwise without prior written permission of the copyright holder. This book is intended for entertainment purposes only and does not imply legal, medical, financial or other professional advice. The reader should seek the help of a competent professional for all matters.

Photo Credits:

All photos are original photos taken or created by the author or rights purchased at Fotolia.com. All rights to appear in this book have been secured.

Some images within this book are either royalty-free images, used under license from their respective copyright holders, or images that are in the public domain. Images used under a creative commons license are duly attributed, and include a link to the relevant license, as per the author's instructions. All Creative Commons images used under the following license. All works in the public domain are considered public domain given life of the author plus 70 years or more as required by United States law.

36 Nursing Cheat Sheets

for Students

NRSNG.com | NursingStudentBooks.com

Jon Haws RN CCRN
Sandra Haws RD CNSC
TazKai LLC

Introduction

First of all . . . THANKS! Thank you for supporting NRSNG.com and for sharing our mission of improving nursing education. My journey into nursing was a long one but I have found it to be a truly rewarding career that allows me to make a difference and have ample family time. I am confident that you will achieve your goals. The fact that you are seeking additional resources to improve your understanding speaks volumes to your dedication.

Second of all, this book is intended to provide you with a quick reference to some of the most needed and most used information for nursing students.

This is not a complete guide to nursing but a simple and compact quick reference to some of the most important information.

As always you should consult institutional policies when it comes to patient care.

Happy Nursing!

-Jon Haws RN CCRN

NRSNG.com | NursingStudentBooks.com

Your Free Gift!

As a way of saying thanks for your purchase, I'm offering a free PDF download:

"63 Must Know NCLEX® Labs"

With these charts you will be able to take the 63 most important labs with you anywhere you go!

You can download the 4 page PDF document by going to NRSNG.com/labs

Table of Contents

Injection Sites (IM)

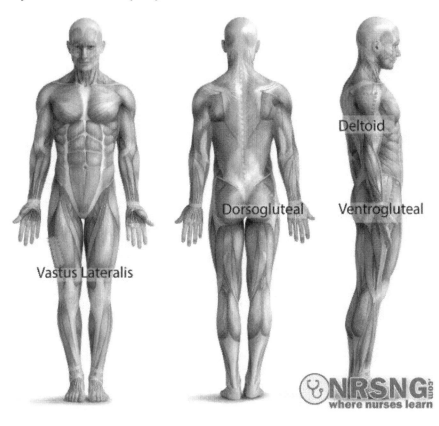

Deltoid

Dorsogluteal

Ventrogluteal

Vastus Lateralis

Common Laboratory Values

Complete Blood Count (CBC) with Differential			
Value	**Abbreviation**	**Unit**	**Normal Range**
Red Blood Cell	RBC	$x10^6$/ml	Male: 4.5 - 5.5 Female: 4.0 - 4.9
White Blood Cell	WBC	cells/mcL	4,500 - 10,000
Neutrophils			54 - 62%
Band Forms			3 - 5% (>8% = left shift)
Eosinophlis			1 - 3%
Basophils			0 - 0.75%
Lymphocytes			25 - 33%
Monocytes			3 - 7%
Platelets	PLT	cells/mcL	100,000 - 450,000
Hemoglobin	Hgb	g/dl	Male: 13.5 - 16.5 Female: 12.0 - 15.0
Hematocrit	Hct	%	Male: 41 - 50 Female: 36 - 44
Mean Corpuscular Volume	MCV	fL	80 - 100
Red Cell Distribution Width	RDW		<14.5

Blood Chemistry (Basic Metabolic Panel) (BMP)			
Value	**Abbreviation**	**Unit**	**Normal Range**
Sodium	Na+	mEq/L	135 - 145
Potassium	K+	mEq/L	3.5 - 5.5
Chloride	Cl-	mEq/L	96 - 108
Glucose	Glu	mg/dL	70 - 115
Calcium	Ca^{2+}	mg/dL	8.4 - 10.2
Creatinine	Cr	mg/L	0.7-1.40
Blood Urea Nitrogen	BUN	mg/dL	7-20

Coagulation Studies

Value	Abbreviation	Unit	Normal
Prothrombin Time	PT	Seconds	11 - 14
Partial Thromboplastin Time	PTT	Seconds	25 - 35
International Normalized Ratio	INR		0.8 - 1.2
Activated Partial Thromboplastin Time	aPTT		1.5 - 2.5

Cholesterol Levels

Value	Abbreviation	Unit	Normal
Cholesterol Total		mg/dL	<200
Low Density Lipoprotein	LDL	mg/dL	<70
High Density Lipoprotein	HDL	mg/dL	<60 optimal
Triglycerides		mg/dL	<150

Arterial Blood Gas

Value	Abbreviation	Unit	Normal
pH	pH		7.35 - 7.45
Partial Pressure of CO_2	pCO_2	mmHg	35 -45
Partial Pressure of O_2	pO_2	mmHg	80 - 100
Bicarbonate	HCO_3	mEq/L	22 - 26
Base Excess	BE	mEq/L	-2 - +2
Oxygen Saturation	SaO_2	%	95 - 100

Blood Gas Analysis

Value	Normal Range	What does it mean?
pH	7.34-7.44	The pH or H+ indicates if a patient is acidemic (pH < 7.35; H+ >45) or alkalemic (pH > 7.45; H+ < 35).
Arterial oxygen partial pressure (PaO2)	75-100 mmHg	A low PaO2 indicates that the patient is not oxygenating properly, and is hypoxemic. (Note that a low PaO2 is not required for the patient to have hypoxia.) At a PaO2 of less than 60 mm Hg, supplemental oxygen should be administered. At a PaO2 of less than 26 mmHg, the patient is at risk of death and must be oxygenated immediately
Arterial carbon dioxide partial pressure (PaCO2)	35-45 mmHg	The carbon dioxide partial pressure (PaCO2) is an indicator of CO2 production and elimination: for a constant metabolic rate, the PaCO2 is determined entirely by its elimination through ventilation.[9] A high PaCO2 (respiratory acidosis, alternatively hypercapnia) indicates underventilation (or, more rarely, a hypermetabolic disorder), a low PaCO2 (respiratory alkalosis, alternatively hypocapnia) hyper- or overventilation.
HCO3–	22–26 mEq/L	The HCO3– ion indicates whether a metabolic problem is present (such as ketoacidosis). A low HCO3– indicates metabolic acidosis, a high HCO3– indicates metabolic alkalosis. As this value when given with blood gas results is often calculated by the analyzer, correlation should be checked with total CO2 levels as directly measured.
Base excess	-2 to +2 mmol/L	The base excess is used for the assessment of the metabolic component of acid-base disorders, and indicates whether the patient has metabolic acidosis or metabolic alkalosis. Contrasted with the bicarbonate levels, the base excess is a calculated value intended to completely isolate the non-respiratory portion of the pH change. There are two calculations for base excess (extra cellular fluid - BE(ecf); blood - BE(b)). The calculation used for the BE(ecf) = cHCO3 - 24.8 +16.2 X (pH-7.4). The calculation used for BE(b) = (1-0.014 x hgb) x (cHCO3 - 24.8 + (1.43 x hgb + 7.7) x (pH -7.4).

Blood Gas Interpretation

Respiratory Acidosis	pH	PaCO$_2$	HCO$_3$
Acute	< 7.35	> 45	Normal
Partly Compensated	< 7.35	> 45	> 26
Compensated	Normal	> 45	> 26
Respiratory Alkalosis			
Acute	> 7.45	< 35	Normal
Partly Compensated	> 7.45	< 35	< 22
Compensated	Normal	< 35	< 22
Metabolic Acidosis			
Acute	< 7.35	Normal	< 22
Partly Compensated	< 7.35	< 35	< 22
Compensated	Normal	< 35	< 22
Metabolic Alkalosis			
Acute	> 7.45	Normal	> 26
Partly Compensated	> 7.45	> 45	> 26
Compensated	Normal	> 45	> 26

Blood Compatibility

Blood Group	Antigens	Antibodies	Can give blood (RBC) to	Can receive blood (RBC) from
AB	A and B	None	AB	AB, A, B, O
A	A	B	A and AB	A and O
B	B	A	B and AB	B and O
O	None	A and B	AB, A, B, O	O

User:Luigi Albert Maria (Own work) [CC BY-SA 3.0 (http://creativecommons.org/licenses/by-sa/3.0)], via Wikimedia Commons

Anticoagulant Therapy

Lab values for individuals on anticoagulant therapy

INR: 2-3 dependant on indication

(http://www.globalrph.com/warfarin_inr_targets.htm)

$$INR = \frac{PT_{test}}{PT_{normal}}$$

Heart Murmurs

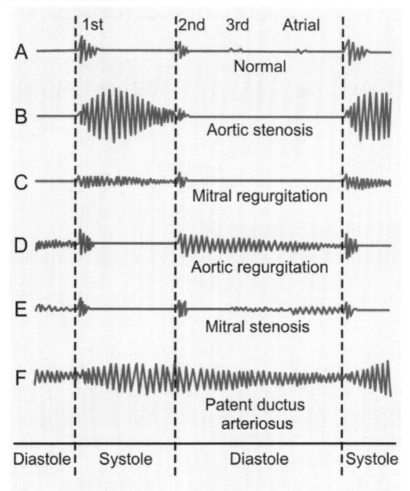

Phonocardiograms from normal and abnormal heart sounds

Glasgow Coma Scale

	1	2	3	4	5	6
Eye	Does not open	Opens to painful stimuli	Opens to voice	Opens spontaneously	N/A	N/A
Verbal	Makes no sound	Incomprehensible sounds	Utters inappropriate words	Confused, disoriented	Oriented	N/A
Motor	No movement	Extension to painful stimuli (decerebrate response)	Abnormal flexion to painful stimuli (decorticate response)	Withdraws to painful stimuli	Localizes to painful stimuli	Obeys commands

Cranial Nerves

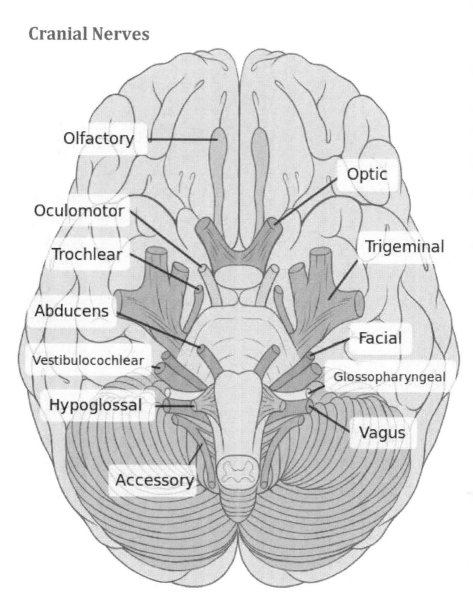

Olfactory

Optic

Oculomotor

Trigeminal

Trochlear

Abducens

Facial

Vestibulocochlear

Glossopharyngeal

Hypoglossal

Vagus

Accessory

Brain_human_normal_inferior_view.svg: Patrick J. Lynch, medical illustrator derivative
work: Beao derivative work: Dwstultz [CC BY 2.5
(http://creativecommons.org/licenses/by/2.5)], via Wikimedia Commons

Wallace Rule of Nines - Burn Severity

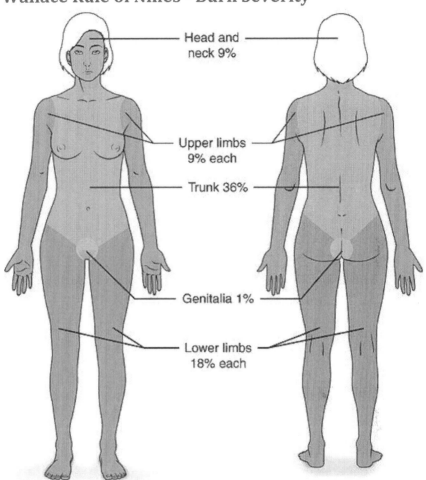

Head and neck 9%

Upper limbs 9% each

Trunk 36%

Genitalia 1%

Lower limbs 18% each

By OpenStax College [CC BY 3.0 (http://creativecommons.org/licenses/by/3.0)], via Wikimedia Commons

Edema Scale

1+: Mild: both feet/ankles

2+: Moderate: both feet, plus lower legs, hands or lower arms

3+: Severe: generalized bilateral pitting edema, including both feet, legs, arms, and face

4+: >30 seconds to rebound

Wigger Diagram

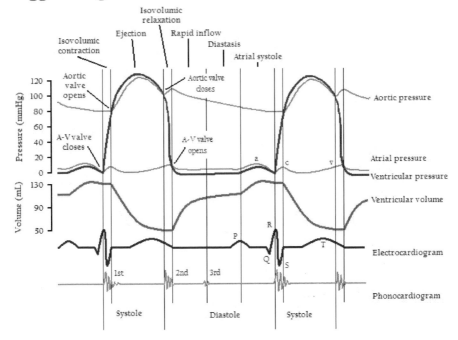

Correspondence between valves, beats, pressures, and sounds within the heart.

Heart Sounds

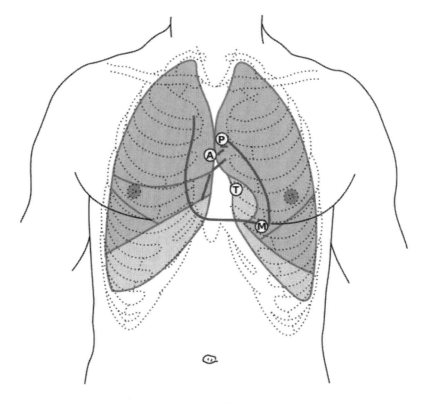

By Madhero88 (Own work Reference netter image) [CC BY-SA 3.0
(http://creativecommons.org/licenses/by-sa/3.0)], via Wikimedia Commons

Locations for listening to heart sounds: **APE To Man**

Normal EKG

P Wave · PR Segment · QRS Complex · ST Segment · T Wave · U Wave · PR Interval · QT Interval

By Derivative: Hazmat2 Original: Hank van Helvete (This file was derived from: EKG Komplex.svg) [CC BY-SA 3.0 (http://creativecommons.org/licenses/by-sa/3.0)], via Wikimedia Commons

12 Lead EKG Placement

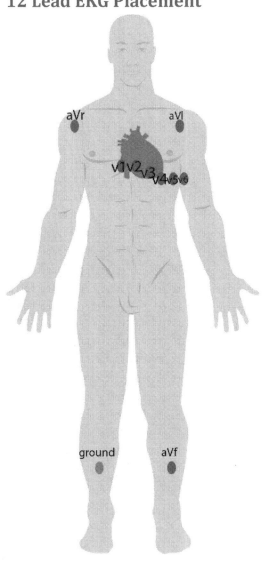

EKG Strip Interpretation

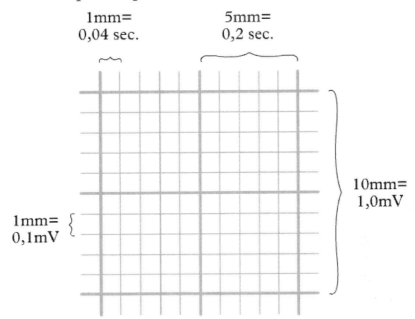

1mm=
0,04 sec.

5mm=
0,2 sec.

1mm=
0,1mV

10mm=
1,0mV

ECGPEDIA.ORG

Abnormal EKG

STEMI V1 - V5 notice the ST elevation in leads V1 - V5

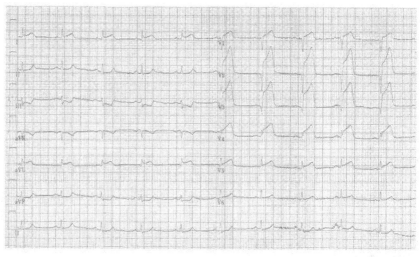

ECG PEDIA.ORG

Ventricular Tachycardia

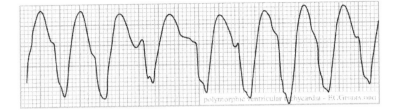

polymorphic ventricular tachycardia - ECGpedia.org

PCV - notice the early ventricular beat

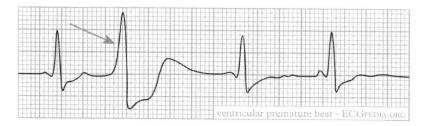

ventricular premature beat - ECGpedia.org

Atrial Flutter

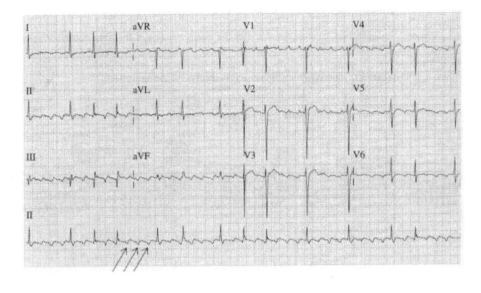

Atrial Fibrillation with RVR

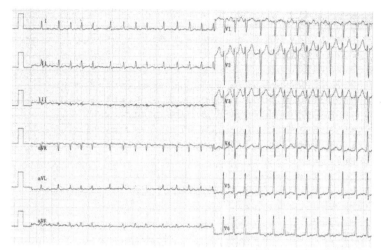

Courtesy of R.W. Koster, MD, PhD   ECG-QUBDIA.ORG
AMC, The Netherlands

5 Lead EKG Placement

White on Right (arm) - Black on Left (arm)
Green on Right (ABD or leg) - Red on Left (ABD or leg)

Mnemonic:
Snow over Trees - Smoke over Fire

Heart Murmurs

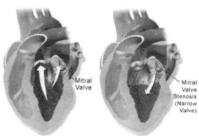

Mitral Valve Regurgitation   Mitral Valve Stenosis

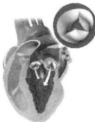
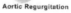
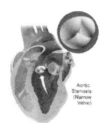

Aortic Regurgitation   Aortic Stenosis

By BruceBlaus. Blausen.com staff. "Blausen gallery 2014". Wikiversity Journal of Medicine.
DOI:10.15347/wjm/2014.010. ISSN 20018762. (Own work) [CC-BY-3.0
[http://creativecommons.org/licenses/by/3.0]], via Wikimedia Commons

	AORTIC	MITRAL
SYSTOLE	OPEN STENOSIS	CLOSED REGURGITATION
DIASTOLE	CLOSED REGURGITATION	OPEN STENOSIS

Shock

The goal of the cardio-pulmonary system is to deliver O2 to the body

Shock is a state of vital organs not receiving adequate O2

3 Main Types of Shock

Hypovolemic - Low volume

Cardiogenic - Broken pump (heart)

Septic - Immune response interferes with vascular tone

Normal Oxygen Delivery System

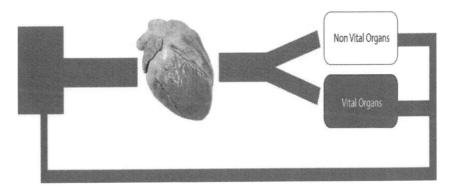

Non Vital Organs

Vital Organs

With each type of shock a different portion of the O2 deliver system is effected:

Hypovolemic - The initial insult is low blood volume

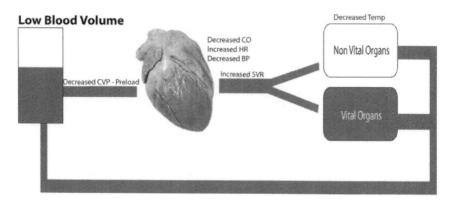

Low Blood Volume

Decreased CO
Increased HR
Decreased BP

Increased SVR

Decreased CVP - Preload

Decreased Temp

Non Vital Organs

Vital Organs

Hypovolemic Shock Stages:

Class I: 500-750 ml loss

Class II: 750-1500 ml loss

Class III: 1500-2000 ml loss

Class IV: >2000 ml

Cardiogenic - Initial insult is pump failure

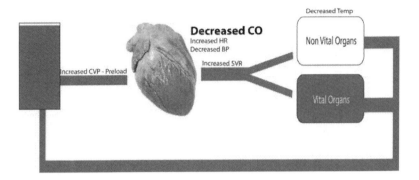

Septic - Immune response (inflammation) initiates systemic vasodilation

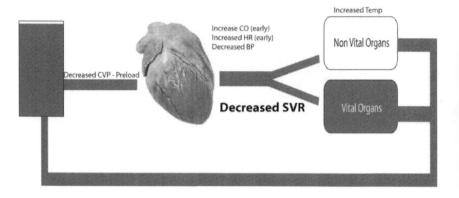

Decreased CVP - Preload

Increase CO (early)
Increased HR (early)
Decreased BP

Increased Temp

Non Vital Organs

Decreased SVR

Vital Organs

Comparison of Different Types of Shock (NOT all inclusive)

	Hypovolemic	Cardiogenic	Septic
CO	↓	↓ Initial Insult	↑ (early)
HR	↑	↑	↑ (early)
SVR	↑	↑	↓ Initial Insult
EF	↑	↓	↓
PAOP (L Atria)	↓	↑	↓
CVP R Preload	↓ Initial Insult	↑	↓
BP	↓	↓	↓
Temp	↓	↓	↑

Hierarchy of O2 Delivery

Nasal Cannula
1 lpm = 24%
2 lpm = 28%
3 lpm = 32%
4 lpm = 36%
5 lpm = 40%
6 lpm = 44%

Simple Face Mask
5 lpm = 40%
6 lpm = 45-50%
7 lpm = 50-55%
8 lpm = 55-60%

Non-rebreather Mask
6 lpm = 60%
7 lpm = 70%
8 lpm = 80%
9 lpm = 90%
10 lpm = close to 100%

Venturi Mask
4 lpm = 24-28%
8 lpm = 35-40%
12 lpm = 50%

Trach Collar
21-70% at 10L

T-Piece
21-100% with flow rate at 2.5 times minute ventilation

CPAP
Positive airway pressure during spontaneous breaths

Bi-PAP
Positive pressure during spontaneous breaths and preset pressure to be maintained during expiration

SIMV
Preset Vt and f. Circuit remains open between mandatory breaths so pt can take additional breaths. Ventilator doesn't cycle during spontaneous breaths so Vt varies. Mandatory breaths synchronized so they do not occur during spontaneous breaths.

Assist Control
Preset Vt and f and inspiratory effort required to assist spontaneous breaths. Delivers control breaths. Cycles additionally if pt inspiratory effort is adequate. Same Vt delivered for spontaneous breaths.

(http://web.missouri.edu/~danneckere/pt316/case/pulm/FiO2.htm)

(http://web.missouri.edu/~danneckere/pt316/case/pulm/FiO2.htm)

http://www.ucdenver.edu/academics/colleges/medicalschool/departments/medicine/intmed/imrp/CURRICULUM/Documents/Oxygenation%20and%20oxygen%20therapy.pdf

Wound (Pressure Ulcer) Staging

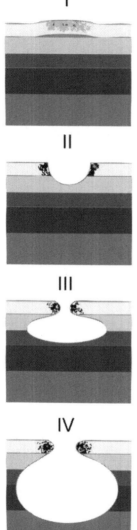

By Nanoxyde [GFDL (http://www.gnu.org/copyleft/fdl.html) or CC BY-SA 3.0 (http://creativecommons.org/licenses/by-sa/3.0)], via Wikimedia Commons

IV Fluid Therapy

One liter of Ringers Lactate solution contains:

130 mEq of sodium ion = 130 mmol/L
109 mEq of chloride ion = 109 mmol/L
28 mEq of lactate = 28 mmol/L
4 mEq of potassium ion = 4 mmol/L
3 mEq of calcium ion = 1.5 mmol/L

One liter of 0.9% Saline contains:

154 mEq of sodium ion = 154 mmol/L
154 mEq of chloride ion = 154 mmol/L

One liter "banana bag" contains 1L of normal saline (sodium chloride 0.9%) with:

Thiamine 100 mg
Folic acid 1 mg
MVI 1 amp (Multivitamin for infusion, 1 ampule)
3 grams of magnesium sulfate

Medication Antidotes

Medication	Antidote
Tylenol	Acetylcysteine (mucomyst)
Potassium	Insulin, $NaHCO_3$, Kayexalate, albuterol
Iron	Deferoxamine
Digoxin	Digiband
Benzodiazepines	Flumazenil (Romazicon)
Magnesium Sulfate	Calcium Gluconate
Opioids	Naloxone (Narcan)
Narcotics	Naloxone (Narcan)
Heparin	Protamine Sulfate
Coumadin	Vitamin K

Insulin Onset, Peak, and Durations

Type of Insulin	Brand Name	Generic Name	Onset	Peak	Duration
Rapid-acting	NovoLog	Insulin aspart	15 minutes	30 to 90 minutes	3 to 5 hours
	Apidra	Insulin glulisine	15 minutes	30 to 90 minutes	3 to 5 hours
	Humalog	Insulin lispro	15 minutes	30 to 90 minutes	3 to 5 hours
Short-acting	Humulin R Novolin R	Regular (R)	30 to 60 minutes	2 to 4 hours	5 to 8 hours
Intermediate-acting	Humulin N Novolin N	NPH (N)	1 to 3 hours	8 hours	12 to 16 hours
Long-acting	Levemir	Insulin detemir	1 hour	Peakless	20 to 26 hours
	Lantus	Insulin glargine			
Pre-mixed NPH (intermediate-acting) and regular (short-acting)	Humulin 70/30 Novolin 70/30	70% NPH and 30% regular	30 to 60 minutes	Varies	10 to 16 hours
	Humulin 50/50	50% NPH and 50% regular	30 to 60 minutes	Varies	10 to 16 hours
Pre-mixed insulin lispro protamine suspension (intermediate-acting) and insulin lispro (rapid-acting	Humalog Mix 75/25	75% insulin lispro protamine and 25% insulin lispro	10 to 15 minutes	Varies	10 to 16 hours
	Humalog Mix 50/50	50% insulin lispro protamine and 50%	10 to 15 minutes	Varies	10 to 16 hours

Source: NIH.gov(http://diabetes.niddk.nih.gov/dm/pubs/medicines_ez/insert_C.aspx)

Common Drug Stems

Source NIH.gov
(http://druginfo.nlm.nih.gov/drugportal/jsp/drugportal/DrugNameGenericStems.jsp)

Stem	Drug Class
-adol or -aldol-	Analgesics
-alol	Combined alpha and beta blockers
-arone	Antiarrhythmics
-aril	Antiviral
-teplase	Enzymes; tissue plasminogen activators
-azepam	Antianxiety
-barb or barb-	Barbituric acid derivatives
-cef	Cephlosporins
-coxib	Cyclooxygenase-2 inhibitors
-cort-	Cortisone derivatives
-conazole	Systemic antifungals
-dil-, dil-, or - dil	Vasodilators
-mycin	Antibiotic
nal-	Narcotic agonist/antagonist
-olol	Beta-blockers
-olone	Steroids
-pamil	Coronary vasodilators
-perone	Antianxiety agents
-pezil	Acetylcholinesterase inhibitors
-pidem	Hypnotics/sedative
-prazole	Antiulcer agent
-pressin	Vasoconstrictors
-pril	ACE inhibitors
-sartan	ARBs
-semide	Diuretic
-sporin	Immunosuppressants
-terol	Bronchodilators
-thiazide	Diuretics
-tricin	Antibiotics
-vir, -vir-, vir-	Antiviral

Common Critical Care Drips

Check with you institutional policies prior to starting or titrating ANY drip

Drug	Brand Name	Dose	Use	Other
Nicardipine	Cardene	5-15 mg/hr	decrease BP	Ca Channel Blocker - Do NOT give with nimotop
Norepinephrine	Levophed	5-30 mcg/min	Increase BP	
Fentanyl	Sublimaze	25-200 mcg/hr	Pain Control	
Propofol	Diprivan	20-200 mcg/kg/min	Sedation	SAT RASS
Versed	Midazolam	1-10 mg/hr	Sedation	SAT RASS
Vasopressin	Pitressin	units/min	DI, Sepsis, hypotension	ADH - Titrate to urine output -Cause decreased Urine Specific Gravity
Heparin		units/kr/hr	Anticoagulation	Draw PTT (blue top)
Insulin		units	Decrease BS	
Neosnyphrine	phenylephrine	40-200 mcg/min	Increase BP	
Dexmedetomidine	Precedex	0.1-0.7 mcg/kg/hr	Sedation	SAT RASS

NRSNG
where nurses learn

Common Light Sensitive Drugs

Partial list of common medications that are light sensitive. Consult drug guide, pharmacist, and institutional guidelines prior to administering any medication.

Acylovir tab
Adrenaline inj
Aminophylline/Theophylline
Amlodipine + HCTZ
Atropine Sulfate inj
Atenolol tab
Ceftriaxone inj
Dexamethasone inj
Diazepam tab/inj
Digoxin
Fluoxetine tab
Furosemide tab/inj
Losartan potassium tab
Metoprolol tab
Nifedipine cap
Naloxone inj
Proporanolol tab
Rifampin tab
Thyroxin tab

Source: (http://www.pharmyaring.com/download/doc100122083450.pdf)

Celsius to Fahrenheit Conversion

Celsius	Fahrenheit
36	96.8
36.1	96.98
36.2	97.16
36.4	97.52
36.5	97.7
36.7	98.06
36.8	98.24
36.9	98.42
37	98.6
37.1	98.78
37.2	98.96
37.4	99.32
37.5	99.5
37.6	99.68
37.8	100.04
37.9	100.22
38	100.4
38.1	100.58
38.2	100.76
38.4	101.12
38.5	101.3
38.6	101.48
38.8	101.84
38.9	102.02
39	102.2
39.1	102.38
39.2	102.56
39.4	102.92
39.5	103.1
39.6	103.28
39.8	103.64
39.9	103.82

40	104
40.1	104.18
40.2	104.36
40.4	104.72
40.5	104.9
40.6	105.08
40.8	105.44
40.9	105.62
41	105.8

Nursing Calculations

$$\frac{Ordered}{Have} = Dose$$

$$\frac{Concentration\ \%}{100} X\ Volume = Dosage\ Amount$$

$$\frac{Volume}{Time} = Flow\ Rate$$

$$\frac{Volume(mL)}{Time\ (minutes)}\ x\ Drop\ Factor\ \left(\frac{gtts}{mL}\right)$$
$$= Flow\ Rate\ (\frac{gtts}{minute})$$

*weight in Kg * Dose per Kg = Required Dose*

$$\frac{weight\ (kg)}{height(meter)^2} = BMI$$

Nursing Math Conversions

1 teaspoon (t) = 5 ml

1 tablespoon (T) = 3 t = 15 ml

1 oz = 30 ml

1 cup = 8 oz

1 quart = 2 pints

1 pint = 2 cups

1 grain (gr) = 60 mg

1 gram (g) = 1,000 mg

1 kilogram (kg) = 2.2 lbs

1 lb = 16 oz

APGAR Scoring

	0	1	2
Appearance	Blue or pale	Blue at extremities, body pink	No cyanosis, body and extremities pink
Pulse Rate	Absent	<100 bpm	>100 bpm
Reflex Irritability	No response to stimulation	Grimace on suction or stimulation	Flexed arms and legs that resist extension
Activity	None	Some flexion	Flexed arms and legs resist extension
Respiratory Effort	Absent	Weak, irregular, gasping	Strong, lusty cry

Breath Sounds

Wheeze or rhonchi	continuous	high (wheeze) or lower (ronchi)	expiratory or inspiratory	whistling/sibilant, musical	asthma, many others
Stridor	continuous	high	either, mostly inspiratory	whistling/sibilant, musical	epiglottitis, foreign body, laryngeal oedema, croup
Inspiratory gasp	continuous	high	inspiratory	whoop	pertussis (whooping cough)
Crackles (rales)	discontinuous	high or low, nonmusical	inspiratory	cracking/clicking/rattling	pneumonia, congestive heart failure

Maslow Hierarchy of Needs

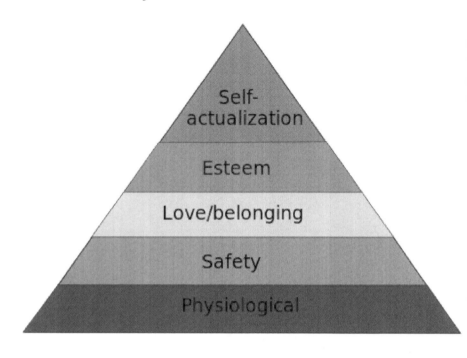

By FireflySixtySeven [CC BY-SA 4.0 (http://creativecommons.org/licenses/by-sa/4.0)], via Wikimedia Commons

Head to Toe Assessment Checklist

Recommended order for head to toe assessment-not intended to be a complete assessment guide.

- o General Assessment
- o Body Structure/Mobility
- o Behavior
- o Health History
- o Vital Signs
  - o Height Weight
  - o Pulse Rate
  - o Respirations
  - o Temperature
  - o Blood Pressure
  - o Pain
- o Integumentary
  - o Inspect: color, moisture, hair, rashes, lesions, pallor, edema
  - o Palpate: temperature, turgor, lesions, edema, texture
- o Scalp
  - o Inspect: shape, symmetry
  - o Palpate: tenderness, deformity
- o Nails
  - o Inspect: shape, color
  - o Palpate: capillary refill
- o Head
  - o Inspect: symmetry, shape, size, uniformity
- o Neck
  - o Inspect: symmetry, lesions, scars
  - o Palpate: tenderness, lymph nodes, thyroid gland, TMJ
- o Eyes

- Inspect: interior and exterior, visual fields, acuity, reflexes
- Ears
  - Inspect: color, shape, symmetry, interior inspection
  - Palpate: tenderness, deformity
- Nose
  - Inspect: shape, symmetry, interior inspection
  - Palpate: frontal sinus, maxillary sinuses
- Mouth and Throat
  - Inspect: exterior and interior
- Thorax and Lungs (anterior and posterior)
  - Inspection: respiration quality, symmetry, deformity, tracheal location
  - Palpation: tenderness, fremitus, chest expansion
  - Percussion: percussive tones, diaphragmatic excursion
  - Auscultation: breath sounds and quality
- Heart and Great Vessels
  - Inspection: jugular venous pulse
  - Palpate: pulses, PMI
  - Auscultate: heart sounds (bell and diaphragm)
- Peripheral Vascular System
  - Inspect: color, edema
  - Palpate: temperature, edema
- Abdomen
  - Inspect: discomfort, uniformity, color, symmetry, scars, hernia, peristalsis, pulsations
  - Auscultate: bowel sounds, bruits
  - Percussion: four quadrants, liver, spleen, renal tenderness

- o Palpation: light to deep, liver, spleen, aorta, rebound tenderness, fluid wave
- o Musculoskeletal
  - o Inspection: asymmetry, deformity, atrophy
  - o Palpation: major joints, tenderness, deformity, range of motion
- o Neurological
  - o Inspect: mental status (health history), cranial nerves, coordination, movement, senses
  - o Palpate: motor strength, muscle tone, reflexes, senses
- o Genitourinary
  - o Inspect: general appearance, lesions, scars
  - o Palpate: breast exam, testicular exam, prostate exam, vaginal exam, Pap smear
- o Lymphatic
  - o Palpate: assess lymph node locations

Adult Vital Signs

HR: 60-100 bpm

RR: 12-20 rpm

BP: <120/<80 mmHg (heart.org)

Temp: 37°C (98.6°F)

Your Free Gift!

As a way of saying thanks for your purchase, I'm offering a free PDF download:

"63 Must Know NCLEX® Labs"

With these charts you will be able to take the 63 most important labs with you anywhere you go!

You can download the 4 page PDF document by going to NRSNG.com/labs

About the Authors

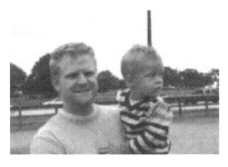

Sick of spending hours and hours trying to find all the information you need for clinical and NCLEX® study? So was I . . . . That's why I created NRSNG.com, a community of nurses and nursing students wanting to jump start their careers.

I am a registered nurse and CCRN on a Neurovascular Intensive Care Unit at a Level I Trauma Hospital. I attended college at Brigham Young University and later received my Nursing degree from Methodist College in Peoria, IL. I also hold a Business Management degree from Touro University.

Professionally, I precept nursing students and new graduate Registered Nurses and work as a charge nurse . . . and love it!

Come visit us at NRSNG.com or check in on Facebook.com/NRSNG.

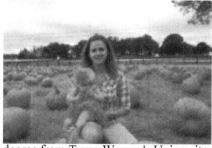

Sandra is a dietitian with one of the largest health care systems in the United States. She works with intensive care patients. She obtained her undergraduate degree from Brigham Young University and her graduate degree from Texas Woman's University. She holds advanced certifications in nutrition support management.

Visit NursingStudentBooks.com to view more books.

Visit NRSNG.com to view our apps, books, videos and more.

40278593R00035

Made in the USA
Lexington, KY
30 March 2015